The Mitochondria Code

Unlocking the Secrets of Cellular Energy

Albert Hazel

Disclaimer: The information in this book is not meant to be used as medical advice; rather, it is meant only for educational reasons. It is not meant to replace expert medical supervision or be used for diagnosis. It is recommended that you discuss any medical problem with a healthcare provider before using any information provided.

The publisher and the author disclaim any liability for any injury allegedly resulting from material found in this book.

Contents

Chapter One

Introduction to Mitochondria

The vital cellular organelles in charge of producing energy are called mitochondria. They have their own genome, which codes for trnas and rrnas required for protein translation, as well as proteins involved in electron transport and oxidative phosphorylation. They are encased in a double-membrane system. In eukaryotic cells, mitochondria are essential for producing metabolic energy. This energy is mostly produced by oxidative phosphorylation, which turns energy from the breakdown of carbohydrates into atp. Because of their distinct genetic makeup and functional properties, mitochondria are essential for the production of cellular energy and may have consequences for a number of illnesses, such as cancer, diabetes, and obesity.

Understanding the function of mitochondria in the cellular energy production process could help us understand the underlying processes of various disorders and potentially lead to the development of novel therapeutic solutions.

The genome of mitochondria is a circular double-stranded DNA molecule that is 16.5 kb in size. It is divided into light and heavy strands according to the nucleotide composition of each strand. Important proteins involved in the respiratory chain, which is fundamental to the process of oxidative phosphorylation, are encoded by this genome. Human health and disease are greatly impacted by the distinct genetic features of the mitochondrial genome, such as its susceptibility to mutations and maternal inheritance. Numerous mitochondrial diseases, which affect energy generation and result in a wide range of clinical symptoms, can be caused by mutations in the mitochondrial genome. Deciphering the composition and operation of the mitochondrial DNA is essential to understanding cellular energy and how it affects human health.

> **Historical Overview**

The powerhouses of the cell, mitochondria, have an interesting past. It is believed that an old symbiotic relationship between an enveloped prokaryote and a nucleated cell gave rise to these organelles. The absorbed prokaryote's offspring eventually gave rise to mitochondria, which gave rise to their distinctive features like a double membrane and their own DNA. The circular, double-stranded DNA molecule that makes up the mitochondrial genome, or mitochondrial DNA (mtDNA), encodes vital proteins needed for the synthesis of energy. The genetic code of the cell's mitochondria is different from its nucleus DNA in a number of ways. Because it raises issues about the origin and significance of this unique characteristic, both creationism and evolutionary biologists have expressed interest in this deviant genetic code. Understanding the genetic and historical characteristics of mitochondria is crucial for understanding how they have influenced the evolution of eukaryotic cells and how they function in the creation of cellular energy.

Richard Altmann initially noticed mitochondria in cells in the late 1800s, which led to their discovery. But the whole understanding of mitochondria's function in energy production did not come about until the 1960s. The electron transport chain in mitochondria creates a proton gradient across the inner mitochondrial membrane, which is then used to manufacture ATP by oxidative phosphorylation. This process was explained by Peter Mitchell's chemiosmotic theory. The subject of bioenergetics was completely transformed by this hypothesis, which also won Mitchell the 1978 Chemistry Nobel Prize. Since then, research on mitochondria has broadened to encompass their function in a number of cellular functions, including the generation of reactive oxygen species, calcium signaling, and apoptosis. The identification of mitochondrial diseases, such as mitochondrial encephalomyopathy and Leigh syndrome, has brought even more attention to the significance of these organelles in human health and illness. A study of the historical background of mitochondria is necessary to appreciate their importance in the synthesis of cellular energy and their effects on human health.

> Importance in Cellular Energy

As the primary source of the chemical energy required to drive the cell's metabolic activities, mitochondria are essential to the creation of energy within cells. Adenosine triphosphate (ATP) is a tiny molecule that stores the energy produced by mitochondria. Nearly all eukaryotic cells have membrane-bound organelles called mitochondria, which have their own genome and a modified genetic code. Here is a summary of the role mitochondria play in cellular energy:

1. Energy production: In eukaryotic cells, mitochondria are the main location of energy generation. They use the process of oxidative phosphorylation to transform the energy obtained from the breakdown of carbohydrates into ATP.

2. Cellular functions: apoptosis, calcium signaling, and phospholipid synthesis are just a few of the cellular tasks that mitochondria are involved in.

3. Regulation of cellular energy production: Since mitochondria are in charge of coordinating cellular energy generation and preserving cellular viability, they are essential to the regulation of cellular energy production.

4. Disease implications: Numerous illnesses, including Parkinson's, heart disease, diabetes, and cancer, have been related to defects in mitochondrial function. The development of possible therapeutic applications and treatments for these disorders

requires an understanding of the role played by mitochondria in the creation of cellular energy.

5. Evolutionary implications: Evolutionary biologists and creationists have been interested in the deviant genetic code found in mitochondria, which is different from the universal genetic code used by most living organisms. This has raised questions regarding the origin and function of this unusual feature.

Mitochondria are essential organelles for the synthesis of cellular energy and are involved in a number of different cellular functions. Their distinct genetic traits and roles have consequences for human health, illness, and the evolutionary history of cellular energy generation.

Beyond just producing energy, mitochondria are also engaged in other crucial cellular processes. They are essential in controlling the process of apoptosis, which controls both cell division and proliferation. Furthermore, calcium signaling—which is necessary for a number of cellular processes, such as the contraction of muscles and the release of neurotransmitters—is centered on mitochondria.

These organelles also contribute significantly to the production of reactive oxygen species (ROS), which have effects on oxidative stress and cell signaling.

The effects of dysfunctional mitochondria are extensive. In addition to the conditions already listed, such as diabetes and Parkinson's, mitochondrial dysfunction has also been linked to age-related decline, cardiovascular disease, and neurodegenerative disorders. It is essential to comprehend the role mitochondria play in cellular energy production as well as their wider effects on cellular function in order to further research and create viable treatments for a variety of human disorders.

Chapter Two

Mitochondrial Structure and Function

Membrane-bound organelles that are present in nearly all eukaryotic cells, mitochondria, are known as the "powerhouses of the cell" because of their crucial function in the production of cellular energy. The majority of the cell's supply of adenosine triphosphate (ATP), the main source of energy for the cell, is produced by these organelles. The inner and outer mitochondrial membranes are divided by an intermembrane space, which defines the double-membrane system that makes up the structure of mitochondria. The electron transport chain and ATP production protein complexes are housed in the many folds known as cristae that the inner membrane generates to enhance its surface area.

Mitochondria are home to their own genome, called mitochondrial DNA (mtDNA), which codes for tRNAs and rRNAs required for protein translation in addition to critical proteins involved in oxidative phosphorylation and electron transport. Different from the nuclear genome, the mitochondrial genome is a circular double-stranded DNA molecule. Because of a certain genetic trait, mitochondria are able to synthesize certain proteins that are necessary for their operation.

The primary job of mitochondria is to produce energy by means of an inner mitochondrial membrane activity known as oxidative phosphorylation. Through a sequence of protein complexes, electrons are transferred throughout this process, producing ATP. Furthermore, mitochondria are engaged in other critical cellular functions such as heme and phospholipid production, apoptosis, and calcium signaling.

A cell's need for energy might affect how many mitochondria it has. For example, mitochondria are highly concentrated in muscle and nerve cells because they use a lot of energy. In addition to producing energy, mitochondria also generate the iron complex required for red blood cells, store calcium ions, and participate in the process that causes cell death.

In conclusion, the role that mitochondria play in supplying energy to cells is closely related to both their structure and function. The majority of the biochemical and physiological functions of the cell are powered by ATP, which is produced exclusively by these organelles. They are also essential for the maintenance of life and the control of numerous cellular processes since they are involved in a broad variety of cellular functions beyond the production of energy.

> Anatomy of Mitochondria

As previously mentioned, eukaryotic cells' cytoplasm contains membrane-bound organelles called mitochondria. Because of their crucial role in the provision of cellular energy, they are frequently referred to as the "powerhouses of the cell." The inner and outer mitochondrial membranes are divided by an intermembrane space, which defines the double-membrane system that makes up the structure of mitochondria. The protein complexes involved in the electron transport chain and ATP generation are housed in the multiple folds known as cristae that the inner membrane creates, increasing its surface area.

The genome found in mitochondria, called mitochondrial DNA (mtDNA), is unique to each mitochondria and codes for tRNAs and rRNAs needed for protein translation as well as critical proteins involved in energy production, such as those needed for the electron transport chain and oxidative phosphorylation. Different from the nuclear genome, the mitochondrial genome is a circular double-stranded DNA molecule. Because of a certain genetic trait, mitochondria are able to synthesize certain proteins that are necessary for their operation.

The primary job of mitochondria is to produce energy by means of an inner mitochondrial membrane activity known as oxidative phosphorylation. Through a sequence of protein complexes, electrons are transferred throughout this process, producing ATP. Furthermore, mitochondria play a role in other critical cellular functions such as heme and phospholipid production, apoptosis, and calcium signaling.

A cell's need for energy might affect how many mitochondria it has. For example, mitochondria are highly concentrated in muscle and nerve cells because they use a lot of energy. In addition to producing energy, mitochondria also generate the iron complex required for red blood cells, store calcium ions, and participate in the process that causes cell death.

To sum up, the structure of mitochondria, featuring their distinct double-membrane configuration and internal cristae, is closely associated with their role in supplying energy to the cell. The majority of the biochemical and physiological functions of the cell are powered by ATP, which is produced exclusively by these organelles. They are essential for the maintenance of life and the control of numerous cellular processes because they are also involved in a broad variety of cellular functions beyond energy production.

Understanding the structure of mitochondria is crucial to comprehending their function in the synthesis of cellular energy. Important aspects of the anatomy of mitochondria include:

1. Dual membrane architecture: The inner and outer mitochondrial membranes of mitochondria, which are divided by an intermembrane gap, make up the double-membrane structure of these membrane-bound organelles. The inner mitochondrial membrane is highly specialized, creating many folds known as cristae that enhance its surface area and contain the protein complexes involved in the electron transport chain and ATP synthesis. The outer mitochondrial membrane is a simple membrane.

2. Cristae: To increase its surface area and give more room for the enzymatic activities involved in energy production, the inner mitochondrial membrane folds several times into what are known as cristae. Protein complexes that are essential to oxidative phosphorylation and energy production, including the ATP synthase complex and respiratory chain enzymes, make up the cristae.

3. Protein complexes: A variety of protein complexes are found in mitochondria and are involved in the ATP synthesis and electron transport chains. These protein complexes, which consist of ATP synthase, cytochrome c oxidase, and

NADH-ubiquinone oxidoreductase, are found in the inner mitochondrial membrane.

4. The matrix of mitochondria: The gel-like material that contains additional proteins and enzymes necessary for the synthesis of energy is called the matrix. It acts as a medium for the chemical reactions that occur inside the mitochondria.

5. DNA from mitochondria: The genome found in mitochondria, called mitochondrial DNA (mtDNA), is unique to each mitochondria and codes for tRNAs and rRNAs needed for protein translation as well as critical proteins involved in energy production, such as those needed for the electron transport chain and oxidative phosphorylation. Different from the nuclear genome, the mitochondrial genome is a circular double-stranded DNA molecule.

Gaining an understanding of the structure of mitochondria is essential to understanding their function in the creation of cellular energy and their involvement in a number of cellular processes, including apoptosis, calcium signaling, and the synthesis of heme and phospholipids.

The production of cellular energy in the form of adenosine triphosphate (ATP) depends on the electron transport chain (ETC), a crucial process that occurs inside the mitochondrial membrane. It is a sequence of chemical molecules and protein complexes that electrons move through in a sequence of redox reactions to release energy. The protein ATP synthase uses this energy to produce a proton gradient, which in turn fuels the synthesis of a significant amount of ATP.

The four primary protein complexes that make up the ETC are cytochrome c reductase (Complex III), succinate dehydrogenase (Complex II), cytochrome c oxidase (Complex IV), and NADH-ubiquinone oxidoreductase (Complex I). The production of ATP is facilitated by the electron transfers and electrochemical gradients produced by these protein complexes.

Protons are pumped across the inner mitochondrial membrane as a result of electron transport via these protein complexes, forming a gradient. In a process known as chemiosmosis, ATP synthase uses this gradient, a type of potential energy, to produce ATP.

An essential part of oxidative phosphorylation, the metabolic process by which cells produce most of their ATP, is the ETC. This activity is critical to the cell's energy requirements and is especially important in cells that require a lot of energy, including muscle and nerve cells, which have a high concentration of mitochondria to meet their needs.

In conclusion, the electron transport chain plays a key role in the creation of cellular energy, and understanding it is essential to deciphering the mechanisms underlying this process as well as how it affects different physiological and cellular functions.

> ATP Synthesis

The process by which adenosine triphosphate (ATP) is created in the mitochondria, the organelles in charge of producing energy within cells, is known as ATP synthesis. The creation of ATP, the principal energy currency of the cell, is necessary for the biochemical and physiological functions of the cell.

The inner mitochondrial membrane is the site of a process known as oxidative phosphorylation, which produces ATP. Through a sequence of protein complexes, electrons are transferred throughout this process, producing ATP. In a process known as chemiosmosis, the energy generated during this process is utilized to establish a proton gradient across the inner mitochondrial membrane, which is subsequently used by the protein ATP synthase to synthesize ATP.

A molecular device called ATP synthase catalyzes the creation of ATP by utilizing the energy contained in the proton gradient. This process's molecular machinery transforms chemical energy into mechanical energy, electrical energy, and finally chemical energy, which is used to create ATP.

For a cell to meet its energy requirements, the process of ATP synthesis is necessary. This is especially true for cells that require a lot of energy, such as muscle and nerve cells, which contain a high concentration of mitochondria. Numerous biological functions, including muscular contraction, nerve impulse transmission, and biosynthesis, are powered by the ATP that mitochondria produce.

To sum up, the synthesis of ATP is an essential step in the production of cellular energy, and comprehending this process is vital to deciphering the mechanisms involved in the production of cellular energy and its influence on many physiological and cellular processes.

Chapter Three

Genetic Blueprint of Mitochondria

Mitochondrial DNA (mtDNA), a circular double-stranded DNA molecule, is the genetic blueprint of mitochondria and is encoded in their own genome. In humans, mitochondria comprise 37 genes that are necessary for proper mitochondrial activity. These genes encode molecules known as transfer RNA (tRNA) and ribosomal RNA (rRNA), as well as enzymes involved in oxidative phosphorylation.

A distinctive feature of mitochondrial DNA is its altered genetic code. This indicates that, in contrast to the universal genetic code utilized by the majority of living things, it employs a distinct set of codons to identify the same set of amino acids. Because it raises issues about the origin and purpose of this unique characteristic, both creationism and evolutionary biologists have expressed interest in this deviant genetic code.

Understanding the mitochondria's function in cellular energy production and how it affects human health requires knowledge of their genetic makeup. Numerous mitochondrial diseases, which affect energy generation and result in a wide range of clinical symptoms, can be caused by mutations in the mitochondrial genome. Understanding the genetic makeup of mitochondria can help one better understand how they function in the synthesis of cellular energy and how that might affect human health.

> Mitochondrial DNA

Mitochondrial DNA, or mtDNA, is a special and important part of cellular genetics and is crucial for the production of cellular energy. In contrast to nuclear DNA, which is inherited from both parents, maternal tDNA is only transferred to her kids. The mitochondria, which are the organelles in a cell that produce energy, contain this genetic material. About 16,500 base pairs make up the human mtDNA, which is home to 37 genes that are essential for regular mitochondrial activity. Instructions for thirteen of these genes code for enzymes involved in oxidative phosphorylation, which produces adenosine triphosphate (ATP), the main energy source for the cell. The molecules that the remaining genes encode, known as ribosomal RNA (rRNA) and transfer RNA (tRNA), are necessary for protein synthesis in the mitochondria.

Recent studies have shown that some mtDNA genetic information can integrate into the nuclear genome in about one out of every 4,000 births. This finding sheds light on the evolutionary history of humans. It has been demonstrated that this process, known as nuclear-embedded mitochondrial DNA sequences, occurs, and scientists are currently investigating the causes of this integration.

Genetics, evolution, and human health are all very interested in mtDNA because of its special properties, which include its maternal inheritance and function in energy production. Deciphering the mysteries surrounding cellular energy generation and its wider consequences for human biology and illness requires an understanding of the structure, function, and heredity of mtDNA.

> Inheritance and Replication

Multiple proteins and enzymes must work in unison to replicate mtDNA, which is a complicated process. While mtDNA replication happens continuously throughout the cell cycle, nuclear DNA replication only happens during the S phase of the cell cycle. To guarantee that the proper amount of mitochondria is maintained within the cell and that the mitochondrial genome is reproduced appropriately, the replication of mtDNA is strictly regulated.

The only way that mtDNA is inherited is through the mother. This makes it special. This indicates that the father does not contribute any mtDNA to the offspring; instead, all offspring inherit it from their mother. Because this form of inheritance makes it possible to track maternal lineages back through time, it has significant implications for population genetics and human evolution research.

In conclusion, mtDNA inheritance and replication are crucial aspects of cellular genetics that are crucial to the supply of cellular energy. Genetics, evolution, and human health are all very interested in mtDNA because of its special properties, which include its maternal inheritance and function in energy production. Deciphering the mysteries surrounding cellular energy generation and its wider consequences for human biology and illness requires an understanding of the structure, function, and heredity of mtDNA.

Chapter Four

Mitochondrial Dysfunction and Diseases

A broad spectrum of disorders resulting from compromised mitochondrial function are together referred to as mitochondrial dysfunction. Environmental causes, genetic mutations, or a mix of the two can induce mitochondrial malfunction. A class of hereditary illnesses known as mitochondrial disorders is caused by abnormalities in nuclear genes or the mitochondrial genome that impact the function of the mitochondria. Although these conditions can affect any organ or tissue in the body, they frequently impact high-energy organs, including the heart, brain, and muscles.

Numerous illnesses, such as cancer, metabolic, cardiovascular, and neurological diseases, have been related to mitochondrial malfunction. For instance, mitochondrial malfunction has been connected to Huntington's disease, Parkinson's disease, and Alzheimer's disease. Furthermore, diabetes, heart disease, and stroke have all been linked to mitochondrial dysfunction.

New diagnostic techniques and possible therapeutic interventions have been developed as a result of research into mitochondrial dysfunction and its role in disease. For instance, the application of mitochondrial replacement therapy, which substitutes healthy mitochondria from a donor for the damaged mitochondria in a patient's cells, is being investigated by researchers. Treatment for diseases associated with dysfunctional mitochondria and other problems related to mitochondria has shown promise with this technique.

In conclusion, the term "mitochondrial dysfunction" is broad and is used to characterize a variety of disorders resulting from compromised mitochondrial activity. A class of hereditary illnesses known as mitochondrial disorders is caused by abnormalities in nuclear genes or the mitochondrial genome that impact the function of the mitochondria. Numerous illnesses, such as cancer, metabolic, cardiovascular, and neurological diseases, have been related to mitochondrial malfunction. New diagnostic techniques and possible therapeutic interventions have been developed as a result of research into mitochondrial dysfunction and its role in disease.

> **Role in Health and Disease**

With their crucial role in the synthesis of cellular energy, mitochondria are frequently referred to as the "powerhouses of the cell." Their primary job is the process of oxidative phosphorylation, which produces adenosine triphosphate (ATP), the cell's energy currency. The majority of physiological and metabolic functions, including growth, mobility, and homeostasis, depend on ATP.

Disturbances in the synthesis of energy, which frequently result from dysfunction in the mitochondria, can cause a variety of illnesses, such as cancer, metabolic disorders, cardiovascular diseases, and neurodegenerative diseases. Due to their high energy requirements, the muscles, heart, and brain are especially susceptible to energy failure, which can result in diseases like stroke, heart disease, Parkinson's disease, and Alzheimer's disease.

There has been a renaissance of interest in the study of mitochondrial function and cellular bioenergetics, as evidenced by publications and activity on the subject. This is because of their functions in apoptosis, the generation of radicals, aging, and illness, in addition to energy metabolism. Beyond producing ATP, mitochondria also play a wide range of other functions, such as acting as hubs for the biosynthesis of lipids, amino acids, and nucleotides.

In conclusion, mitochondria play a variety of roles in both health and sickness. Although their role in energy production is the main reason for their recognition, they are important for many cellular functions and have a big impact on human health. Uncovering the mysteries of cellular energy and its wider influence on human biology and disease requires a thorough understanding of the intricacies of mitochondrial activity.

> Common Mitochondrial Disorders

A collection of clinically diverse and heterogeneous inborn errors of metabolism that arise from compromised mitochondrial activity are known as mitochondrial diseases. Mutations affecting mitochondrial function in nuclear genes or the mitochondrial genome (mtDNA) can be the cause of several illnesses. Because of some peculiarities of mitochondrial genetics, diagnosis can be difficult even with an increasing understanding of the genetic causes of this class of illnesses. A molecular diagnosis is still elusive for many people with mitochondrial diseases, which can be difficult to diagnose. Nearly 290 genes have been found to be the genetic origins of various illnesses, but our knowledge of how these flaws result in cellular malfunction and organ pathology is still developing.

Any organ or tissue in the body can be impacted by mitochondrial diseases, but they frequently affect the brain, heart, and muscles, which are among the organs that use a lot of energy. Numerous clinical symptoms, such as those of neurodegenerative illnesses, cardiovascular diseases, metabolic disorders, and cancer, are linked to these conditions. The brain, heart, and muscles are among the organs with the highest energy requirements, making them especially susceptible to energy failure. Over time, this vulnerability can lead to the onset of many diseases.

Understanding the effects of mitochondrial abnormalities on human health and developing viable diagnostic and treatment strategies depend heavily on the research on these disorders. There are continuous multicenter international clinical trials underway for primary mitochondrial diseases, despite the absence of FDA-approved medicines at this time. Furthermore, the discovery of novel therapeutic targets and the advancement of cutting-edge technologies are improving our knowledge of the pathways essential for the synthesis of cellular energy, which could result in the creation of fresh approaches to treatment.

Chapter Five

Unlocking the Mitochondrial Code

The genetic information included in the mitochondrial DNA (mtDNA) and responsible for producing the proteins and enzymes needed to produce energy within cells is known as the mitochondrial code. 90% of the energy in a cell is produced by double-membrane organelles called mitochondria in the form of ATP. Despite not being completely understood, the mechanism of mitochondrial ATP generation has been the focus of extensive research, and understanding of this essential energy activity is still advancing.

The 37 genes that make up the mitochondrial genome are unique in that they are inherited from the mother and are necessary for proper mitochondrial function. These genes can become mutated to cause mitochondrial diseases, which can affect any organ or tissue in the body but are most commonly found in the brain, heart, and muscles, which are high energy-consuming organs. Numerous clinical symptoms, such as those of neurodegenerative disorders, cardiovascular diseases, metabolic disorders, and cancer, are linked to these conditions.

Understanding the mechanisms behind mitochondrial function and how they affect human health requires a thorough understanding of the mitochondrial code and its function in cellular energy production. Genetics, evolution, and human health are all very interested in mtDNA because of its special properties, which include its maternal inheritance and function in energy production. Uncovering the mysteries of cellular energy and its wider influence on human biology and disease requires an understanding of the intricacies of mitochondrial function.

To sum up, the genetic information included in the mitochondrial DNA and responsible for producing the proteins and enzymes needed for the synthesis of cellular energy is known as the mitochondrial code. Understanding the mechanisms behind mitochondrial function and how they affect human health requires a thorough understanding of the mitochondrial code and its function in cellular energy production. The domains of genetics, evolution, and human health are all very interested in mtDNA because of its special properties.

> Current Research and Discoveries

The peculiar properties of mitochondrial DNA (mtDNA) and its function in the synthesis of cellular energy have been clarified by recent studies. Known as the "powerhouses of the cell," mitochondria are double-membrane organelles that produce 90% of the energy in a mammalian cell as adenosine triphosphate (ATP) via the oxidative phosphorylation (OXPHOS) process. They are inherited from their mothers and have their own DNA, which is circular, close-stranded, and double-stranded. It differs from nuclear DNA. Only 37 genes, comprising two ribosomal RNA (rRNA) subunits, 22 transfer RNA (tRNA) genes, and 13 genes encoding protein subunits, including the enzyme complex OXPHOS, are found in the tiny (16.5 kilobase pairs) human mtDNA. Numerous mitochondria are found in each cell, and within each of these mitochondria are several copies of mtDNA. These copies can be found in all mtDNA copies (homoplasmy) or in a subset of all copies (heteroplasmy). Challenges in studying mtDNA include the wide variability of clinical symptoms, the non-specific nature of many phenotypes, and the poorly known links between genotype and phenotype. On the other hand, mtDNA sequencing is an essential tool for detecting mutations in order to research the genome, find new variants, and diagnose clinical diseases. Genetics, evolution, and human health are all very interested in mtDNA because of its special properties, which include its absence of introns, maternal inheritance, multiple copy numbers per cell, complicated heteroplasmy, and threshold effect. Uncovering the mysteries of cellular energy and its wider influence on human biology and illness requires a thorough understanding of the mitochondrial code and its function in cellular energy generation. Current investigations, like the one that was just released in PLOS Biology, are helping to clarify the pathways that are essential for producing cellular energy and may also point to new targets for pharmaceuticals. Addressing typical energy issues in cells and creating new treatments for illnesses linked to energy failure, such as mitochondrial disorders, depend on this research.

> Potential Therapeutic Applications

The genetic information included in the mitochondrial DNA (mtDNA) and responsible for producing the proteins and enzymes needed to produce energy within cells is known as the mitochondrial code. Known as the "powerhouses of the cell," mitochondria are double-membrane organelles that produce 90% of the energy in a mammalian cell as adenosine triphosphate (ATP) via the oxidative phosphorylation (OXPHOS) process. They are inherited from their mothers and have their own DNA, which is circular, close-stranded, and double-stranded. It differs from nuclear DNA. Only 37 genes, comprising two ribosomal RNA (rRNA) subunits, 22 transfer RNA (tRNA) genes, and 13 genes encoding protein subunits, including the enzyme complex OXPHOS, are found in the tiny (16.5 kilobase pairs) human mtDNA. Numerous mitochondria are found in each cell, and within each of these mitochondria are several copies of mtDNA. These copies can be found in all mtDNA copies (homoplasmy) or in a subset of all copies (heteroplasmy). Challenges in studying mtDNA include the wide variability of clinical symptoms, the non-specific nature of many phenotypes, and the poorly known links between genotype and phenotype. On the other hand, mtDNA sequencing is an essential tool for detecting mutations in order to research the genome, find new variants, and diagnose clinical diseases. Genetics, evolution, and human health are all very interested in mtDNA because of its special properties, which include its absence of introns, maternal inheritance, multiple copy numbers per cell, complicated heteroplasmy, and threshold effect. Uncovering the mysteries of cellular energy and its wider influence on human biology and illness requires a thorough understanding of the mitochondrial code and its function in cellular energy generation. Current investigations, like the one that was just released in PLOS Biology, are helping to clarify the pathways that are essential for producing cellular energy and may also point to new targets for pharmaceuticals. Addressing typical energy issues in cells and creating new treatments for illnesses linked to energy failure, such as mitochondrial disorders, depend on this research.

Chapter Six

Interplay with Cellular Processes

The domains of human health, evolution, and genetics are all very interested in how the mitochondrial code interacts with cellular functions. Mitochondria are essential for the provision of energy within cells and are closely associated with a number of biological functions, including apoptosis, metabolism, and aging. The synthesis of proteins and enzymes necessary for the synthesis of cellular energy occurs in the organelles, which have their own genomes with altered genetic codes.

According to recent studies, mitochondrial transcription and translation are critical for the oxidative phosphorylation (OXPHOS) system's biogenesis, which produces ATP and the RNA primers required to start mtDNA replication. The OXPHOS system requires the coordinated expression of genes encoded by the mitochondrial and nuclear genomes in order to function properly. The regulation of mitochondrial function and cellular energy generation depends on the interaction between the nuclear and mitochondrial genomes.

Beyond producing ATP, mitochondria also play a wide range of other functions, such as acting as hubs for the biosynthesis of lipids, amino acids, and nucleotides. They are signaling centers that control differentiation, vitality, and death, as well as the integration of the anabolic and catabolic metabolisms. Since mitochondria cannot be created from scratch, they must undergo continuous quality assurance and regeneration via the process of mitotic budding.

Understanding the mechanisms of mitochondrial activity and their consequences for human health requires an understanding of the interactions between the mitochondrial code and cellular processes. Genetics, evolution, and human health are all very interested in mtDNA because of its special properties, which include its absence of introns, maternal inheritance, multiple copy numbers per cell, complicated heteroplasmy, and threshold effect. Uncovering the mysteries of cellular energy and its wider influence on human biology and disease requires a thorough understanding of the intricacies of mitochondrial function.

> Mitochondria and Metabolism

Mitochondria are essential for the provision of energy within cells and are closely associated with a number of biological functions, including apoptosis, metabolism, and aging. The manufacture of proteins and enzymes necessary for the synthesis of cellular energy is carried out by the organelles, which have their own genomes with altered genetic codes. Understanding the mechanisms of mitochondrial activity and their consequences for human health requires an understanding of the interplay between the mitochondrial code and cellular functions.

The hubs of cellular metabolism, mitochondria coordinate a wide range of metabolic processes vital to human health. Together, the genes encoded by the mitochondrial (mtDNA) and nuclear (nDNA) genomes are needed for the coordinated expression of the oxidative phosphorylation (OXPHOS) system, which produces ATP. Not only is mtDNA transcription vital for the biogenesis of the OXPHOS system, but it also produces the RNA primers required to start mtDNA replication.

Beyond producing ATP, mitochondria are essential for the biosynthesis of nucleotides, amino acids, and lipids. They are signaling centers that control differentiation, vitality, and death, as well as the integration of the anabolic and catabolic metabolisms. Since mitochondria cannot be created from scratch, the budding of mitochondrial components allows for continuous quality monitoring and regeneration of the organelles.

Understanding the mechanisms behind mitochondrial activity and how they affect human health requires a thorough understanding of the function of mitochondria in cells. Genetics, evolution, and human health are all very interested in mtDNA because of its special properties, which include its absence of introns, maternal inheritance, multiple copy numbers per cell, complicated heteroplasmy, and threshold effect. Uncovering the mysteries of cellular energy and its wider influence on human biology and disease requires a thorough understanding of the intricacies of mitochondrial function.

> Mitochondria-Cell Nucleus Communication

An essential component of cellular function is the exchange of information between the mitochondria and the cell nucleus. Through the process of oxidative phosphorylation (OXPHOS), mitochondria produce adenosine triphosphate (ATP), which is essential for the provision of energy within cells. Coordinated expression of the genes encoded by the nuclear and mitochondrial genomes is necessary for this process. Retrograde signaling is the continuous transmission of molecular signals by mitochondria to the nucleus, indicating their metabolic state and activity. In response to alterations in mitochondrial activity or cellular stress, these signals have the ability to modify the expression of nuclear genes, especially those related to mitochondrial function.

The regulation of mitochondrial function and cellular energy generation depends on the interaction between the nuclear and mitochondrial genomes. A number of transcription factors go to the nucleus upon activation by changes in mitochondrial activity, including Sp1, SIRT3, and GSP2. These transcription factors target nuclear genes and modify the transcription of genes involved in mitochondrial function based on the molecular signals produced by the mitochondria. This two-way communication is essential for the preservation of cellular homeostasis and is involved in many other cellular functions, such as the biology of muscle cells.

An active and crucial mechanism for controlling cellular metabolism and energy production is communication between the nucleus and mitochondria. Additionally, it is essential for cellular homeostasis maintenance and adaptability to stress. Deciphering this communication is essential to understanding cellular energy and its wider effects on human biology and illness. Genetics, evolution, and human health are among the subjects that are very interested in mtDNA due to its special properties and interactions with the nuclear genome.

Chapter Seven

Future Directions in Mitochondrial Research

Future directions in mitochondrial research include investigating the possibility of using mitochondrial gene therapy to treat diseases related to the mitochondria, figuring out how neurodegenerative disorders cause dysfunction in the mitochondria, and creating plans to improve mitochondrial function in order to improve cellular health. In mitochondrial research, some of the main topics of interest are:

1. Gene therapy: One possible treatment option for mitochondrial illnesses is the development of gene therapy techniques. This includes repairing mutations in the mitochondria and reestablishing mitochondrial function through the use of genome editing tools like CRISPR-Cas9.

2. Mitochondrial dynamics: To learn more about how mitochondria adjust to alterations in cellular demand and respond to stress, researchers are examining the processes of mitochondrial biogenesis, maintenance, and quality control. With this understanding, initiatives to increase cellular health and mitochondrial function can be developed.

3. Mitochondrial role in neurodegenerative disorders: Research on how mitochondria function is essential to understanding the onset and course of neurodegenerative diseases like Alzheimer's, Parkinson's, and Huntington's. In order to enhance mitochondrial function and reduce symptoms, this

entails investigating the processes underlying mitochondrial malfunction in various illnesses and creating viable treatment interventions.

4. Mitochondrial transcription and translation: An important area of study in mitochondrialogy is the control of mitochondrial transcription and translation. Scholars are currently engaged in efforts to get a deeper comprehension of the processes governing the expression of mitochondrial genes and the variables impacting the stability and functionality of mitochondrial proteins.

5. Mitochondrial interplay with cellular processes: An essential component of cellular activity is the interaction of the nuclear and mitochondrial genomes. Scholars are currently examining the mechanisms governing mitochondrial function as well as the effects of dysfunctional mitochondria on cellular functions, including differentiation, apoptosis, and vitality.

By concentrating on these next avenues for mitochondrial research, scientists hope to solve the mysteries surrounding the synthesis of cellular energy and create viable treatment plans for illnesses involving malfunctioning mitochondria.

> Emerging Technologies

Novel tools in the field of mitochondrial research are creating new opportunities to unlock the mysteries of cellular energy production. Among these technologies are a few:

1. CRISPR-Cas9: In mitochondrial illnesses, this novel gene editing technology is being used to repair mutations in the mitochondria and restore mitochondrial function. Researchers may potentially develop novel treatment approaches for mitochondrial illnesses by using CRISPR-Cas9 to target particular mitochondrial genes and alter their DNA.

2. High-throughput sequencing: Large-scale lists of the genes that regulate mitochondrial activity and energy production can now be produced by researchers thanks to cutting-edge sequencing technologies like next-generation sequencing. This method may help identify new therapeutic targets

while also advancing scientific understanding of the processes essential for cellular energy production.

3. Mitochondrial transcription and translation: A more thorough investigation of mitochondrial transcription and translation is being conducted using emerging technologies. Scholars are presently examining the processes that govern the expression of mitochondrial genes and the variables that impact the stability and functionality of mitochondrial proteins.

4. Mitochondrial interplay with cellular processes: New technologies are enabling researchers to examine how the nuclear and mitochondrial genomes interact, offering new perspectives on the mechanisms governing mitochondrial function and the effects of dysfunction on cellular processes, including differentiation, apoptosis, and vitality.

Through the use of these cutting-edge technologies, scientists are able to better understand how cells produce energy and create possible treatment plans for illnesses involving malfunctioning mitochondria.

> Implications for Medicine and Beyond

Recent discoveries in the field of mitochondrial science have important ramifications for medicine and other fields. Researchers are learning more about the molecular mechanisms underlying a number of diseases, including heart failure, neurodegenerative disorders, and disorders involving the mitochondria. This is being accomplished by uncovering the mysteries surrounding cellular energy. This information may help identify novel pharmacological targets and spur the creation of creative treatment approaches.

Understanding the regulation of mitochondrial function and its effects on cellular functions is being greatly aided by research on transcription and translation inside the mitochondria and the interaction between the nuclear and mitochondrial genomes. This information is essential for the creation of new instruments, materials, and understanding for human mitochondrial research and animal models with translational relevance. Furthermore, advances in modeling and intervention techniques are opening doors for the discovery of novel therapeutic targets and the clarification of the pathways connecting the production of energy, ROS, and fuel choice with the myriad other functions of mitochondria.

Moreover, cutting-edge tools for studying mitochondria, like high-throughput sequencing and CRISPR-Cas9, are creating new opportunities for deciphering the mechanisms behind cellular energy production. These technological advancements are giving scientists the means to identify genes that control energy and create viable treatment plans for illnesses involving malfunctioning mitochondria.

In conclusion, there are significant ramifications for medicine and other fields from the latest developments in mitochondrial research. This research is opening doors for the creation of novel treatment approaches and the discovery of new pharmacological targets by illuminating the molecular processes that control cellular energy generation and the function of mitochondria in a variety of disorders. Significant progress in the treatment of heart failure, neurological diseases, and mitochondrial abnormalities could result from this, ultimately enhancing human health and quality of life.

> **Conclusion**

In conclusion, research on the mitochondrial code and how it affects the synthesis of cellular energy is a fast-growing topic that will have a big impact on medicine and other fields. The peculiarities of mitochondrial DNA and how they interact with other cellular functions, such as metabolism, apoptosis, and aging, have been clarified by recent studies. The regulation of mitochondrial function and cellular energy generation depends on the interaction between the nuclear and mitochondrial genomes. Cutting-edge technologies like high-throughput sequencing and CRISPR-Cas9 are creating new pathways for deciphering the mysteries of cellular energy generation and creating viable treatment plans for disorders involving dysfunctional mitochondria. Future directions in mitochondrial research include investigating the possibility of using mitochondrial gene therapy to treat diseases related to the mitochondria, figuring out how neurodegenerative disorders cause dysfunction in the mitochondria, and creating plans to improve mitochondrial function in order to improve cellular health. By concentrating on these next avenues for mitochondrial research, scientists hope to solve the mysteries surrounding the synthesis of cellular energy and create viable treatment plans for illnesses involving malfunctioning mitochondria.

- **Summary of Key Insights**

The topic of studying the mitochondrial code and its function in the creation of cellular energy is one that is rapidly developing and has important applications in medicine and other fields. The peculiarities of mitochondrial DNA and how they interact with other cellular functions, such as metabolism, apoptosis, and aging, have been clarified by recent studies. The regulation of mitochondrial function and cellular energy generation depends on the interaction between the nuclear and mitochondrial genomes. Cutting-edge technologies like high-throughput sequencing and CRISPR-Cas9 are creating new pathways for deciphering the mysteries of cellular energy generation and creating viable treatment plans for disorders involving dysfunctional mitochondria. Future directions in mitochondrial research include investigating the possibility of using mitochondrial gene therapy to treat diseases related to the mitochondria, figuring out how neurodegenerative disorders cause dysfunction in the mitochondria, and creating plans to improve mitochondrial function in order to improve cellular health. By concentrating on these next avenues for mitochondrial research, scientists hope to solve the mysteries surrounding the synthesis of cellular energy and create viable treatment plans for illnesses involving malfunctioning mitochondria. Recent developments in mitochondrial research have broad consequences for medicine and other fields. This research is opening doors for the creation of novel treatment approaches and the discovery of new pharmacological targets by illuminating the molecular processes that control cellular energy generation and the function of mitochondria in a variety of disorders. Significant progress in the treatment of heart failure, neurological diseases, and mitochondrial abnormalities could result from this, ultimately enhancing human health and quality of life.

- **Outlook for Mitochondrial Research**

The topic of studying the mitochondrial code and its function in the creation of cellular energy is one that is rapidly developing and has important applications in medicine and other fields. The peculiarities of mitochondrial DNA and how they interact with other cellular functions, such as metabolism, apoptosis, and aging, have been clarified by recent studies. The regulation of mitochondrial function and cellular energy generation depends on the interaction between the nuclear and mitochondrial genomes. Cutting-edge technologies like high-throughput sequencing and CRISPR-Cas9 are creating new pathways for deciphering the mysteries of cellular energy generation and creating viable treatment plans for disorders involving dysfunctional mitochondria. Future directions in mitochondrial research include investigating the possibility of using mitochondrial gene therapy to treat diseases related to the mitochondria, figuring out how neurodegenerative disorders cause dysfunction in the mitochondria, and creating plans to improve mitochondrial function in order to improve cellular health. By concentrating on these next avenues for mitochondrial research, scientists hope to solve the mysteries surrounding the synthesis of cellular energy and create viable treatment plans for illnesses involving malfunctioning mitochondria. Recent developments in mitochondrial research have broad consequences for medicine and other fields. This research is opening doors for the creation of novel treatment approaches and the discovery of new pharmacological targets by illuminating the molecular processes that control cellular energy generation and the function of mitochondria in a variety of disorders. Significant progress in the treatment of heart failure, neurological diseases, and mitochondrial abnormalities could result from this, ultimately enhancing human health and quality of life.

Reference

Anderson, S., Bankier, A. T., Barrell, B. G., de
Bruijn, M. H., Coulson, A. R., Drouin, J., ... &
Young, I. G. (1981). Sequence and organization of
the human mitochondrial genome. Nature,
290(5806), 457-465.

DiMauro, S., & Schon, E. A. (2003). Mitochondrial
respiratory-chain diseases. New England Journal of
Medicine, 348(26), 2656-2668.

Gorman, G. S., Chinnery, P. F., DiMauro, S., Hirano, M., Koga, Y., McFarland, R., ... & Turnbull, D. M. (2016). Mitochondrial diseases. Nature Reviews Disease Primers, 2, 16080.

Lightowlers, R. N., & Chrzanowska-Lightowlers, Z. M. (2008). Human mitochondrial disease: Leber's hereditary optic neuropathy. Cold Spring Harbor perspectives in biology, 4(12), a011247.

Nunnari, J., & Suomalainen, A. (2012). Mitochondria: in sickness and in health. Cell, 148(6), 1145-1159.

Taylor, R. W., & Turnbull, D. M. (2005). Mitochondrial DNA mutations in human disease. Nature Reviews Genetics, 6(5), 389-402.

Vafai, S. B., & Mootha, V. K. (2012). Mitochondrial disorders as windows into an ancient organelle. Nature, 491(7424), 374-383.

Wallace, D. C. (2005). A mitochondrial paradigm of metabolic and degenerative diseases, aging, and cancer: a dawn for evolutionary medicine. Annual review of genetics, 39, 359-407.

Wallace, D. C. (2010). Mitochondrial DNA mutations in disease and aging. Environmental and molecular mutagenesis, 51(5), 440-450.

About the Author

Albert Hazel emerges as a multifaceted professional, seamlessly blending his expertise as a medical researcher with a passion for literary expression. With nearly a decade devoted to medical research, Hazel has delved deep into the complexities of the healthcare landscape, making significant contributions to the advancement of scientific knowledge and innovation.

For over eight years, Albert Hazel has been at the forefront of medical research, focusing on pivotal areas that shape the future of healthcare. His dedication to exploring novel therapies, understanding disease mechanisms, and enhancing patient outcomes reflects a commitment to making a lasting impact in the field.

Beyond the realm of medical research, Hazel channels his creativity and insights into writing, establishing himself as a distinguished book author. His literary works resonate with a blend of scientific rigor, compelling narratives, and a keen understanding of human experiences within the healthcare context. Through his writings, Hazel invites readers on enlightening journeys, fostering a deeper appreciation for the intricacies of medicine and the human spirit.

Albert Hazel's unique blend of medical research and literary exploration exemplifies an interdisciplinary approach to knowledge dissemination. By intertwining scientific expertise with compelling storytelling, he bridges the gap between complex medical concepts and broader audiences, fostering awareness, understanding, and engagement.

Throughout his career, Albert Hazel's contributions have extended beyond traditional boundaries, encompassing both scientific advancements and literary enrichment. His ability to synthesize intricate research findings into accessible narratives underscores a commitment to education, advocacy, and the broader dissemination of knowledge.

In the intricate tapestry of healthcare and literature, Albert Hazel stands as a beacon of innovation, insight, and inspiration. Through his dedicated research endeavors and captivating literary works, he continues to shape conversations, spark curiosity, and leave an indelible mark on both the scientific and literary landscapes.